Oil For The Tin Man

Awaking The Heart

- Paul F. Davis -

:

Men are often overwhelmed with many daily demands and roles placed upon them: operating as sons, brothers, friends, husbands, fathers, employees, business owners, managers, community leaders, athletic coaches, priests, prophets, politicians, peacemakers and much more. Like the tin man in the film *The Wizard of Oz*, men are in need of the oil of the Holy Spirit to lubricate and liberate them when they feel weary in well doing.

Jesus and the apostle Paul exhorted humanity to NOT be restless, careful and overly concerned about earthly things (Matthew 6:25-33), but rather in all things with prayers and supplications; make our requests made known to God and thereafter let the peace of God, which surpasses the mind's understanding, rule our hearts and minds in Christ Jesus (Philippines 4:6-7). In fact, God through king Solomon exhorts us to "guard our heart, which is the wellspring of life" (Proverbs 4:23). So valuable is the heart, that when patients experience heart failure, they pay cardiologists over $100,000 dollars in the United States for surgery to remove the blockages and restore their blood's circulation to sustain the flow of life within their body. Ohio's Cleveland Clinic, according to data from the U.S. Centers for Medicare & Medicaid Services, charged patients $106,385 in 2013, for heart surgery.

https://www.bloomberg.com/news/articles/2013-07-28/heart-surgery-in-india-for-1-583-costs-106-385-in-u-s-

Remember the extraordinary value of your heart, as the wellspring of life (personal and professional) and the source of all inspiration, creativity, ingenuity and passion to propel your life forward. The Word of God is a lamp to illuminate and lighten our steps and direct our path forward (Psalm 119:105), while imparting health to our mortal bodies and making us whole entirely body-mind-spirit (Proverbs 4:20-22; 1Thessalonians 5:23).

God promises in His Word to anoint us with "fresh oil" (speaking of the blessed Holy Spirit) to energize, empower and equip us for greatness, success and victory over every battle we face daily (see Psalm 92:10). Like a unicorn God will anoint and raise us up to excel and prevail in life for His glory, if we remain humble, attentive and dependent upon His input, guidance and divine impartation for momentum and supernatural strength.

Yet only as we awake and come to ourselves, acknowledge and see our weakness and need; can we truly recognize how deeply and desperately we need the assistance and intervention of God daily to empower and uphold us as we endure and go through many challenges in life.

Only when the prodigal son, who foolishly departed from his father and squandered his substance gotten hastily and prematurely, lost everything and came to himself (Luke 15:13-19); could he then humble himself, get brutally honest, grow in self-awareness and intelligently return to his father in his despair and desperation (knowing he was far better with his father than left to his own demise).

The word "anoint" in the Hebrew means to massage and paint. Interestingly, our wonderful, loving and most kind heavenly Father wants to give us a rub down and massage the kinks out of our life (heart, soul and body) by the supernatural power of the Holy Spirit. Having lived and traveled throughout many nations in Asia, where often there are three or four spas on nearly every street; I have often indulged myself and fell asleep on many massage tables for two hours getting a deep tissue muscular massage, while snoring and slobbering all over myself. Yet when I awoke and heard, "Massage finished sir." I can definitely confess I felt more relaxed, emotionally and physically relieved of unnecessary tension, mental turmoil, burdens of the day and week, and delivered from the emotional baggage (heavy, soul crushing conversations and lingering afflictions of less than encouraging people and their unkind conversations) and many distasteful mental memories. Truly the body and mind are interconnected whether we want to admit it or not. What we do with the one truly and always affects the other.

I know some of you are thinking in your carnal mind, I got a happy ending. Not at all, because I don't find joy in strangers for profit touching me like that and the few times when therapists offered on their own initiative (prompted by their selfish monetary motives) to provide additional services for some extra money (trying to negotiate a deal and up sell me on the massage table); I adamantly refused and never returned thereafter to that spa (because those type of therapists usually are just posers and aren't properly trained in deep tissue muscular massage). It's as frustrating as going to a church with good intentions hoping to hear from and receive a blessing from God; but instead you get spiritually violated, never fed any substance to enrich your soul, and only told the importance of giving an offering to make the church bank account grow.

As for my massage preferences, I also don't like to get a woman bigger than me, who gets joy in twisting me like a pretzel (as some Thai massage therapists who want to take me through a yoga workout simultaneously, while giving me a massage). I prefer to do my yoga outside the spa and not during a massage, as I separate the two (similar to a sauna and yoga, as I'm not much of a fan of hot yoga, unless that is the only form of yoga offered and taught in town as was the case when I lived in Laredo, Texas - near the border of Mexico - for a few months). In China during reflexology, some older massage therapists found joy in digging their knuckles into my the bones of my feet and applying pressure to the extent of causing me pain (that lasted for two to three weeks whenever I stood and tried to walk).

This being said, there are many different types of massage techniques (as there are different churches and ministers, some not truly representing the heart, compassion, love and life of God to humanity). Ministers and spiritual teachers practice the art of ministry differently, think differently according to their theological training and mentors (as massage therapists operate differently, and sometimes try to match their approach and therapy to the client or patient they are serving).

Hawaiians use a lomi-lomi technique with long strokes. Japanese use shiatsu style deep tissue, applied pressure massage into critical and vital areas, spots and points throughout the body. Koreans implement and use soft black stones when performing a massage. The Swedish give more of a sports massage. The Indonesians use a Balinese type of massage, somewhat similar to a Swedish massage. The Russians use some unique techniques to relieve tension and knots within the muscles (as they locate one problematic point or place in the body and grind into it with their finger tips in a circular motion in hopes of relieving the tension, liberating the built up blockages and restoring blood circulation). In India, I once watched a Pastor friend of mine from the United States receive a massage (not my favorite technique) wherein he chuckled and said he felt like he was being buffed like a car.

That being said massage therapists throughout the world operate differently, use various techniques, and strive to accomplish different things. As for God Almighty who made the human spirit, soul, and body; He knows best what is needed for and by each individual (God being all-knowing and all-powerful; omniscient and omnipotent). Therefore God by the power of the Holy Spirit, also known as the spirit of love (Romans 5:5) and who Jesus called the Comforter (John 14:26), is able to intervene and work magnificently and miraculously in your life. It can happen while you are sleeping and God visits you during the night with dreams and visions (Acts 2:17), what Bishop T.D. Jakes calls "pillow talk" as God speaks to us during our times of deep sleep. Such is the language and one of the many methods of the Holy Spirit and Almighty God to comfort, counsel, touch, transform, grab, get through to, arrest, shake and awake people.

God takes away burdens and destroys yokes of bondage and oppression by the entrance of the blessed anointing of the Holy Spirit (see Isaiah 10:27). The Holy Spirit removes the demonic spirit of bondage that torments and oppresses people with fear (Romans 8:15) to set the captives free and enable humanity to joyfully experience liberty (Luke 4:18). Because where the Spirit of the Lord God Almighty is, there will be glorious liberty and freedom (2Corinthians 3:17). When the touch of God comes to you and the Holy Spirit begins to apply divine pressure to the troublesome areas and sore spots of your life, the light and glory of God's supernatural power will drive away darkness and transform you in a deep, irresistible and undeniable way.

The Wizard of Oz is a fantastic children's movie that depicts three different types of men: a lion without courage, a scarecrow without a brain, and a tin man without a heart. Therefore all Dorothy wanted to do is run away, she finding no peace or contentment with such characters (though she tried desperately to continually comfort and emotionally carry them to the best of her ability).

The Wizard of Oz is "a 1939 American musical fantasy film produced by Metro-Goldwyn-Mayer, currently distributed by Warner Bros. Pictures. Widely considered to be one of the greatest films in cinema history, it is the best-known and most commercially successful adaptation of L. Frank Baum's 1900 children's book *The Wonderful Wizard of Oz*. The movie was directed primarily by Victor Fleming (who left production to take over the troubled production of Gone with the Wind). The film stars Judy Garland as Dorothy Gale alongside Ray Bolger, Jack Haley, Bert Lahr" (Wikipedia).

"Characterized by its legendary use of Technicolor, fantasy storytelling, musical score, and memorable characters, the film became an icon of American popular culture. It was nominated for six Academy Awards, including Best Picture, but lost to Gone with the Wind, also directed by Victor Fleming. It did win in two other categories: Best Original Song for "Over the Rainbow" and Best Original Scoreby Herbert Stothart. While the film was considered a critical success upon release in

August 1939, it failed to make a profit for MGM until the 1949 re-release" (Wikipedia).

"The 1956 television broadcast premiere of the film on the CBS network reintroduced the film to the public; according to the Library of Congress, it is the most seen film in movie history. It was among the first 25 films that inaugurated the National Film Registry list in 1989. It is also one of the few films on UNESCO's Memory of the World Register. The film is among the top ten in the BFI list of the 50 films you should see by the age of 14" (Wikipedia).

What was it about this film that so captivated and resonated with American and international audiences around the world? What was it about the cast of characters and screenwriting that captivated and intrigued viewers? What about the characters' dilemmas and challenges could we somehow relate to and empathize with as they struggled and worked through their inner issues (which we ourselves can identify with and relate to)? Let us examine a song below, which was sung by the tin man to further help us understand and relate to his inner world.

The tin man sang a revealing song in which he opened up his soul and shared his inner feelings and thoughts, which I will now share here below. A person's favorite song, or one they deeply identify with, embrace and express at a certain season of their life often shows what is truly going on within them. This is why it is important for us to take time to truly listen to people; probe and dig deeper beneath the surface to genuinely get to know them.

Interestingly, before the tin man sang his heartfelt song "if I only had a heart," he says sighs in relief before putting the ax down saying, "I've been carrying this ax for ages."

An ax is used to cut things down and sometimes as a weapon of defense. Thus perhaps the tin man had endured turbulence in life wherewith he had to defend and protect himself with the ax. Such painful experience may have hardened him and caused him to always have his ax and guard up against enemies, evildoers and anyone who might have harmed him.

As one who was thrown into an oxygen tent the first thirty days of my life after birth, raised by my maternal grandparents (my deceased mother having been an alcoholic and drug addict, before being killed by an 18 year old drunk driver), then experienced child abuse under my father and stepmother who worked me like a slave from my youth, endured two failed marriages (the first due to an adulterous affair and the second when my Canadian wife refused to leave America to live with me overseas in Asia for work) and brutal divorces causing me to lose my homes and be left to fight and figure out where I would live and how to survive in this cruel world; I understand how the tin man felt having his ax up always and being continually on guard to protect and defend himself (living in the midst of uncertainty, unsure who you can trust after having been betrayed by those you love, and agonizing to struggle to survive daily with little joy along the way and few friends to enjoy life with who truly understand and appreciate you).

Tin Man (song)

When a man's an empty kettle

He should be on his metal,

And yet I'm torn apart.

Just because I'm presuming

That I could be kind of human,

If I only had a heart

I'd be tender - I'd be gentle

And awful sentimental

Regarding love and art.

I'd be friends with the sparrows

And the boys who shoots the arrows

If I only had a heart.

Picture me - a balcony.

Above a voice sings low.

Dorothy

Wherefore art thou, Romeo?

Tin Man

I hear a beat....How sweet.

Just to register emotion, jealousy - devotion,

And really feel the part.

I could stay young and chipper

And I'd lock it with a zipper,

If I only had a heart.

I commend the tin man for his transparency, honesty, humility and self-awareness. Truly self-awareness is half of the battle, because once a man awakens to who he is and gets brutally honest with himself; thereafter he can acknowledge his strengths, weaknesses, and needs to strategize to how to go about attending to them and transforming his life for the better.

Thankfully, we have a Father in heaven who gives us spiritual vision and songs of deliverance (Acts 26:19; Psalm 32:7) to enable us to see clearly and lift us up to where we belong. Truly as I have experienced in my own heart, soul and body; the anointing of the Lord can heal you within, awaken your heart to the beauty of life and the purity of purposeful living, break toxic entanglements and addictions easily, and energize you entirely spirit-mind-body (read Isaiah 10:27). Moreover once living in, with and on you; the power of the Holy Spirit can inwardly restrain, comfort, counsel, teach, lead and guide you (read John 14:16-17,26; Acts

1:8; 1John 2:27; Zechariah 4:6; John 16:13; Galatians 5:22-25).

Here are a few of my favorite songs pertaining to the oil of the Holy Spirit, the anointing of God for humanity that can love, liberate and lift us to new heights and levels in life.

The Anointing of the Lord

Breaks the yoke of bondage

The anointing of the Lord

Sets the captives free

The anointing of the Lord

Brings rivers in the dessert

The anointing of the Lord

Is raining down on me.

Sweet Holy Spirit

Sweet heavenly dove

Flow like a river

Filling us with your love

And for these blessings

We lift out hearts in praise

And without a doubt we'll know

That we have been revived

When we have left this place.

Anointing, Fall on Me!

Anointing, fall on me!

And let the power of

The Holy Ghost

Fall on me

Anointing fall on me!

Breathe on me!

Breathe on me!

Holy Ghost power

Breathe on me

Yesterday's gone

Today I'm in need

Holy Ghost power

Breathe on me.

Which of the three men are you in the Wizard of Oz? Are you like the lion who lacks courage, the scarecrow lacking a brain, or the tin man missing a heart? Of course the irony in the movie is all three characters already possessed in some form or fashion that which they sought to acquire, it being hidden within them.

Gideon in the Bible was no different, he being fearful and afraid, when God visited him and called Gideon "a mighty man of valor" (Judges 6:11-16). Thus often what we most need is recognition and affirmation to awaken the greatness within us. As a prophetic preacher and worldwide motivational speaker, this is what I do traveling across the globe to awaken and empower people to be their best, transcend their circumstances and past tragedies and traumas, be transformed, arise with courage, vision and faith and boldly and triumphantly step into greatness. Contact me (RevivingNations@yahoo.com) to visit and speak in your city.

Sometimes we get a chip on our shoulder, by reason of past rejection, hurts, wounds and pain we have endured, wrestled with within and had to overcome (sometimes for a lifetime). Legendary basketball great Michael Jordan spoke of his high school basketball coach (during his hall of fame induction speech) who benched him in high school and didn't believe in his abilities. Yet that rejection quite possibly was what angered and drove Jordan to work harder, prove himself, excel in the NBA and become the star we know and admire today.

Therefore thank God for your haters and those who belittle and reject you, because they too are part of the perfecting and maturation process by which God develops your character and energizes you with anger to work harder and be your personal best.

Yet these many tests, continually and persistently overcoming and dealing with rejection, once internalized can (if we are not careful, alert and aware) become a toxic identity that pollutes us within and preprograms us for dysfunction to sideline and derail our present, progress and future.

For example a chip on the shoulder can motivate you to excel as an athlete, but may not help you relationally in marriage or socially when interacting with and seeking to connect and collaborate with others (also a hindrance potentially in the business world).

A chip on the shoulder, originating from insecurity and/or rejection, can lead to you self-sabotaging relationships as you fear ultimately and eventually being hurt; and therefore strive to prematurely sever the relationship (in a toxic attempt to guard your heart from what you perceive, and often falsely so, to be an inevitable hurtful breakup, as your toxic negative beliefs influence your thinking and behavior, invade and pollute your present healthy and meaningful relationship to confirm and affirm your messed up limiting beliefs to justify your foul thoughts, unbelieving actions and confirm what you perceive will ultimately and eventually happen - as you tell yourself you are preparing and protecting yourself from future and foreseeable heartache, a breakup and disaster relationally).

Moreover carrying a chip on your shoulder all of the time is mentally and emotionally exhausting. When basketball great Lebron James won his first NBA championship playing for the Miami Heat, Lebron was asked during the postgame interview: "What made this season different than last year?" (The previous season Lebron's team the Miami Heat made it to the championship tournament, but lost.)

Lebron said this (which I will never forget): "Last year, I played with hate, as I felt I had to prove myself. Whereas this year I played with love." Playing with love thus enabled Lebron to be more relaxed, comfortable in his own skin, focus on his teammates and the group dynamic of the game and the interdependence of the team sport; unlike the preceding year where mentally and emotionally Lebron let the media and fans get to him (some questioning his ability), his reaction to which put the spotlight and attention on himself, which did not serve him well as a person, athlete, teammate and team leader. The inner shift however from hate to love enabled Lebron to be free, focused, more present on the court, excel at the team sport, and lead his team to a championship.

When people are so full of themselves they cannot see and recognize the value of others (or their affect on others), sometimes they need someone to get in their face, usually a friend or a person they love, respect and trust; to shake, awake and tell them to snap out of it and get a grip. Basketball superstars Kobe Bryant and Shaquile O'Neal while playing together on the Los Angeles Lakers had some animosity and hostility brewing between them for a while. It eventually manifested in a brief fight in which a couple punches were thrown before the fight was quickly broken up by players and coaches.

A godly rebuke and confrontation is what the Bible calls "excellent oil" (Psalm 141:5); that which every tin man needs to lubricate their metal arms, legs and joints so they don't get hard and stiff, but can remain flexible and able to move.

Excellent oil in the form of a rebuke is a true manifestation and expression of love (Proverbs 27:5) that will be character building and strengthen a person if they will take off the mask, lay down their pride, dare to listen and reflect on that which is genuinely being said. The alternative and opposite, which most people do around high rolling celebrities and stars, is to always flatter them and kiss their butt continually telling them how great they are (and never pointing out any of their flaws).

Of course we all love praise, affirmation, recognition and to feel good about ourselves. Yet some destructive tendencies, habits, mannerisms and patterns if not confronted and corrected can prove to be harmful, destructive and deadly to our personal well-being, relationships, family, business and beyond.

The Bible says a lying tongue can provide a false sense of certainty and set people up for affliction to be later experienced and flattery works ruin to a person (Proverbs 26:28), corrupting them and making them feel too high-minded and elevated to a place they cannot sustain, the air being thin the higher you climb up the mountain of a great peak and summit.

Certainly it takes focus to envision and see the mountain tops and courage to dare to climb and ascend higher than most dare to go in life.

Undoubtedly every man has degrees of courage, levels of intelligence, and glimpses of his heart throughout his life experience. Yet simultaneously, along a man's lifelong journey; he also will see unpolished and unrefined aspects of his character in situational circumstances that reveal aspects of his inner nature that fall short and lack courage, mindfulness and heart.

Thankfully, all human beings have a wonderful, merciful, and tender Creator who presides over the living and the dead; He being able to touch, transform and save us to the uttermost no matter how undone we see ourselves to be.

The Bible declares God the Father through Jesus Christ can save humanity from the uttermost depths of despair, isolation, agony, chaos, uncertainty, fearfulness, ignorance, and heartlessness. God Almighty took a fearful man named Gideon and made him a mighty warrior, a man named Moses who stuttered and struggled to talk and made him a deliverer and the leader of his people, and a heartless religious murderous zealot by the name of Saul and supernatural touched and transformed him to become the apostle of grace known as Paul who would extend a message of hope to humanity that would transcend generations and reverberate throughout the ages (as the nasty, heartless murderer named Saul would become the apostle Paul and go on to write two-thirds of the New Testament, the Holy Bible that Christians and spiritual seekers across the globe read for faith, hope, love, divine direction and supernatural connection with their Creator).

Each character in *The Wizard of Oz* was awakened to what they truly possessed inwardly when the wizard gave the scarecrow a diploma (symbolizing his intelligence), the lion was given a medal (symbolizing courage) and the tin man was given a ticking heart-shaped watch (to help him visualize and remember he does have a heart). Each gift helped each character (the lion, scarecrow and tin man respectively) see the attributes they sought were already within themselves.

This is often the irony and paradox of life, in that when we see ourselves to be weak and lacking; it is then when actually we are most strong, because we are humble, self-aware and yet bravely willing to walk by faith into the unknown as we step into greatness and believe that which we think and perceive we lack will be awakened and arise within us along our journey, or be added to us serendipitously along the way as we trust our Creator and the universe to conspire to give us what we desire (or orchestrate situations to enable us to see what we seek is simultaneously and supernaturally seeking us, hoping to circumstantially position us and give us opportunities to be turned inside out and discover who we really are as we arise to the occasion and boldly stand forth in the opportunities in front of us).

It is then we can truly stand tall as we awaken to and suddenly see we do have courage (childlike faith and a willpower to boldly enter the unknown and believe for the best), intelligence (emotional intelligence often being far superior to mental knowledge and wisdom), and heart (compassion, passion, affection and tenderness for other humans and animals alike here on earth suffering, coexisting and seeking to survive in similar fashion as we ourselves).

When the wizard in the film offers to take Dorothy and Toto home to Kansas in his hot air balloon, he then reveals that he too is from Kansas. The wizard formerly worked at a carnival when a tornado brought him to the Emerald City. He was offered and accepted the job as wizard due to hard times in his own life, which remind us that fathers too suffer (as does even God Almighty our heavenly Father, who suffers and agonizes over His children and their disobedient wayward hearts that separate them from Him at times until they come to their senses - like the lion, scarecrow and tin man - retain their true authentic identity and return home within their hearts).

As Dorothy and the Wizard prepared to depart and return home, Dorothy's dog Toto, distracted by a cat, leapt from Dorothy's arms (symbolizing how life's distractions often beyond our control continually leap at us and seek to turn our attention and affection away from that which is truly important). Thus one of the biggest battles in life is to fight for our focus and continually pursue that which is important, rather than pursuing distractions and diversions. In other words, when a snake bites your loved one, will you pursue and seek to kill the venomous serpent, or move quickly to get your beloved to the hospital to prevent the spread of infection and death? Where is your focus - saving and improving life, or chasing and killing demons and poisonous monsters? Before seeking to do both, make sure your priorities are in proper alignment, because often you must only choose one of the important options; your choice determining who and what will live and die. A bad choice and wrong pursuit could result in you or your beloved dying. Therefore be smart, alert and aware before moving hastily and emotionally. Know who you are, what you are about, establish your priorities, and remain focused.

In the film "The Wizard of Oz," as Dorothy pursued Toto and put on her ruby slippers (which she was told had the power to return her to Kansas if she tapped her heels together three times while saying "There's no place like home"), upon following the instructions Dorothy thereafter woke up in her bedroom surrounded by her family and friends, including her beloved dog Toto.

Although everyone dismissed Dorothy's adventure as a dream, it was indeed an enlightening one and not surprising since God truly does speak to humanity while we sleep often times (Acts 2:17); visions and dreams being types and shadows that depict in internal imagery our inner struggles and often provide divine direction and illumination to light our road and pathway ahead.

Thus there are many takeaways from the beautiful film, the main themes to me being self-discovery and the pursuit of manhood, dignity, affirmation, love, recognition and a place of belonging which we all call "home" (no matter where geographically that may be or lead us). Home is a place where we are known, not merely by name, but inwardly and celebrated wholeheartedly, loved unconditionally and cared for despite our own shortcomings, setbacks, hang ups, mess ups, mistakes and failures. Thus it is unconditional love, undying faith, and joyful hope that sets the soul free and enables us to live wholeheartedly and freely be (and therein are we most exuberant, at peace and happy).

As we renew our minds with God's Word (Romans 12:1-2) and recognize we were created in God's image (Genesis 1:26-28) we access our divine nature in Christ (2 Peter 1:4) and become a powerful and unstoppable force for good in the earth as we keep our eyes lifted up unto heaven where our help comes from (Psalm 121:1-2).

As the wizard (who admitted he was "not a very good wizard" ha-ha) said, "Every creature has a brain," but those in pursuit of learning attend universities to earn diplomas of graduation affirming thereafter their intellect. Therefore the "wise" wizard gave the scarecrow a degree, an honorary ThD (thinkology), a self-made diploma from a bogus university he made up in his mind, in order to get the scarecrow to believe in himself. It worked as the scarecrow was very proud of himself.

To the lion, the "wizard" told him not to "confuse courage with wisdom," reminding the lion military heroes annually dress up in their formal military uniforms decked out with all of their war medals to parade their heroism down the city streets to remind others of their greatness. Yet "they have no more courage than you have," according to the wizard, "but they have a medal." Therefore the all wise "wizard" conferred on the lion a medal of honor "for meritorious conduct, extraordinary valor, conspicuous bravery against wicked witches." The wizard awarded the lion the triple cross. Upon receipt and hearing such accolades, the lion beamed and was glowing from ear to ear, his countenance bright and radiant (now believing in himself and feeling unstoppable). Thus the lion became a member of "the legion of courage" (as the wizard kissed him on both cheeks and acknowledged his bravery).

The lion overwhelmed with joy never looked so happy and nearly cried with joy overflowing within him, upon hearing such gracious words of praise and adoration, he happily replied with gratitude, "I'm speechless."

This is what we all need from someone and sometimes such words come not from a spouse, parent or family member, but possibly a teacher, friend, or someone in the community. Nevertheless once heard, we feel recognized, loved, affirmed and rise up within to do great things and be our best.

As for the tin man, whom the "wizard" called his "galvanized friend" and reminded him regarding the heart (which the tin man thought he did not possess); "you want a heart, but don't know how lucky you are not to have one."

Indeed sometimes being a bit heartless or hardened by life's tough and turbulent circumstances is a survival mechanism that puts iron in our soul, toughens us to endure and overcome hardships, and press through the pressures of life and not be overcome or undone by them. Nevertheless we all deeply yearn within to possess and manifest heart, show love and kindness to others. Nobody wants to go through life like the wretched, miserable Grinch who rejected every social invitation and was incapable of lightening up, taking a day off work, and celebrating Christmas. The Bible tells us the true desire of a man is showing kindness (Proverbs 19:22).

Thus outward parades of masculinity and competitive virility for show ultimately are attempts for the male to get the female and thereafter be able to let down his guard, take of his armor and mask, and show love and kindness to his damsel (whether in distress or simply in need of love and rest).

Truly the stronger we are, the more gentle we can afford to be. The wiser and smarter we are, the more understanding with others in life we should be as we patiently walk alongside them and seek to teach them what we know to lessen their load, help guide and direct them to paths of peace and prosperity, and befriend them along the way as we display kindness and give assistance.

The wise wizard said, "Hearts will never be practical until they can be made unbreakable." Nevertheless the tin man replied, "but I still want one." The essence of the message here is when you have a heart, the danger is living from the heart is wrought with disappointment as your heart gets disappointed and people fail to live up to your expectations. However living with heart provides a full emotional and sensory experience whereby one can truly feel and enjoy life. Otherwise without heart a person lives like a robot, merely doing things, but never connecting deeply and genuinely with people.

The wise wizard told the tin man: "Back where I come from there are those (philanthropists) who do good deeds all day long and their hearts are no bigger than yours, but they have one thing you haven't got - a testimonial. Therefore in consideration of your kindness, I take pleasure at this time in presenting you a small token of our esteem and affection."

As the wizard gave the tin man a necklace with a red heart, he wisely said to him: "Remember my sentimental friend, a heart is not judged by how much you love, but by how much you are loved by others."

The wisdom of the "wizard" of Oz is quite unique in that he was able to discern the true motivation, deep inclinations and inner yearnings of the scarecrow, lion and tin man. Each deeply yearned for and craved recognition in some way. The scarecrow wanted a brain, the lion courage and the tin man a heart.

The wizard knew the scarecrow, lion and tin man already possessed all of these; but lacked self-awareness because they were looking for the approval and recognition of others (to thereby feel secure in themselves as to what they possessed and expressed).

Never wait for others to identify, recognize and affirm you. In fact if you do, you may wait your whole lifetime and go without it (and live empty and be miserable the entire time while waiting for the accolades and praise of men).

Instead be free to be who you are. Live authentically and freely express yourself, despite those who ignore and fail to recognize you, and despite those who misinterpret, falsely label, belittle and criticize you (sometimes because of their own jealousy, insecurity, and timidity).

Jesus (God manifest in the flesh to help, heal, love, liberate and lift humanity) came to earth first and foremost to heal the brokenhearted and bind up their inner wounds (see John 1:1,14; Luke 4:18). Thus God Almighty in heaven above can feel our pain and heartache (Hebrews 4:15), as we dwell on earth and suffer within (beyond the human eyes of others around about us). Though we tell our friends, classmates and coworkers all is well and carry on with a brave smile (sometimes plastic, other times trying to fake it until we make it); God in heaven knows fully when we hurt and suffer within miserably.

Thankfully Jesus, the rejected and crucified Christ (Isaiah 53), understands pain and suffering immensely and fully; He having been spoken to with nasty words, beaten and whipped like a criminal, and had His face spat on with shame and disgrace by those who falsely accused and reviled Him in public contempt for all to see. Nevertheless wonderful and merciful Jesus forgave all His accusers and abusers freely and wholeheartedly, saying "Father, forgive them; for they do not know what they are doing" (Luke 23:34).

We too must be heavenly minded and see humanity through the eyes of God in order to be able to grasp a higher perspective, see clearly, move forward accurately, relate to others correctly, and navigate our way through life carefully and precisely to avoid the landmines and pitfalls laid out to snare and trap us along the way.

My former Pastor in New York, Bernard Jordan said, "Prayer changes things, beginning with you." To modernize and contextualize the concept, allow me to use a present day example.

Like Boeing recently learned with malfunctions in their airplane software, if incorrectly programmed and warped within, their planes (no matter how beautifully built and regardless of the huge sum of money spent to construct them) will go awry and have fatal crashes despite their pilots good intentions to get to the passengers to their desirable destination.

Sometimes internally we are stuck on stupid and full of ourselves, being snared in a stronghold of pride; thinking ourselves to always be right and irrefutable. Such a perverse mindset sets us on a collision course with others and a path of eventual destruction (as we forget to be mindful of human beings and the world which we together share and all depend to survive and live). Multinational companies that develop hastily and haphazardly disregarding the environment, public health and safety; such corporations will soon self-destruct by reason of their selfish approach to development and blatant disregard of corporate social responsibility and the importance of sustainable development.

In such times of mental anguish, stubbornness and defiance; God often tries to wake us up through situational circumstances and orchestrating interactions with others (sometimes similar to ourselves). God's hope therein and thereby is that we can come to our senses, awake and see ourselves as we truly are (broken, undone, arrogant and often overcome). In the Bible the deceiver Jacob (Genesis 27:1-37) had to meet up with a deceptive man by the name of Laban, who upon deceiving Jacob regarding full and fair compensation for labor done (Genesis 31:3-7), quickly opened Jacob's eyes to the nature of himself and the tendency of humanity to lie, cheat and steal without a God consciousness, fear of deity and morality.

Sometimes when we are deeply entrenched in a wrong mindset, ideology, or are just plain stuck on stupid arrogant defiance; God Almighty in His infinite mercy and loving kindness will meet humanity in the night during times of deep sleep to speak to them and work in the hidden man of the heart (see Job 4:13; Acts 2:17). This is why God gave Jacob the deceiver a dream of blessings from heaven descending upon him (Genesis 28:12) to change Jacob's perspective, inner nature, and the way he related to others (reminding Jacob that God was his Source and Provider). Thereafter Jacob could more easily cope and rest with those in his midst lying, deceiving and stealing from him;

because Jacob knew Almighty God had his back and was looking out for him.

The peace of God surpasses understanding (Philippines 4:7) and enables you to sleep happily and rest in the midst of a storm. Jesus did not worry and concern Himself with storms in His midst, His heart instead being fixed on His heavenly Father; whom He knew would protect and look out for and after Him. Thus in the midst of a violent storm, Jesus kicked back and took a nap (Mark 4:37-39).

Likewise God promises in His Word to keep us in "perfect peace" when we keep our mind and heart on Him (Isaiah 26:3). The key to balancing the hostilities of the natural world externally and the peace of God internally is to see what is going on around you, but be governed and led by what God says and is reiterating and directing within you.

We have to become comfortable with being in overwhelming situations beyond our control and above our heads; that is above and beyond our mental and physical abilities in and of ourselves to fix and resolve the situations (Ezekiel 47:1-5). This is where God Almighty has called us to go, dwell, live and thrive on a daily basis; in hostile situations above and beyond us. Because when man's ability ends, there God's ability can begin to show up and show off (to show Himself strong) if you are willing to give God the glory when He gives you a triumphant victory.

God supernaturally and skillfully, being able to uniquely relate with humanity and their own distinct individuality, thought processes and manner of communication; speaks during deep sleep (sometimes repeatedly until a person finally gets and understands what God is saying) whereby they can perceive and begin to understand the divine message, as God opens their ears, eyes, heart and inwardly imparts and seals His divine instruction within (Job 33:14-16).

God works wonderfully on humanity by putting them into a "deep sleep" during which time God can supernaturally intervene and speak to the unconscious and subconscious mind. God put the first man Adam in a deep sleep (Genesis 2:21), during which time God stole one of Adam's ribs to make for him a wife and helper by the name of Eve.

God spoke to Abram in a dream (Genesis 15:11-13) prior to changing his name to Abraham (Genesis 17:4-6); after which time God established His covenant with Abraham, making him a father of many nations, caused him to be exceedingly fruitful, the father of faith (Romans 4:16) and many nations, and a patriarch to a lineage of future kings.

God performs pillow talk on people supernaturally while they sleep peacefully and rest. Our beloved heavenly Father spoke to the prophet Daniel during his deep sleep, God giving Daniel a dream and insight regarding the end times (see Daniel 8:17-19). Daniel even felt the touch of God in the midst of his sleep, as God Almighty set him upright (Daniel 10:8-10).

Jesus had twelve disciples He called to be apostles, whom He ministered to extensively and attempted to train in the ways of God and ministry. Like most organizations and companies, Jesus too had His stars and others who were a bit slow to catch on. Peter, James and John ascended with Jesus to the mountain of transfiguration (Matthew 17:1-3). Peter could not keep his mouth shut long enough to discern the intention of God, before he tried to label and direct it. Thankfully, God the Father intervened and spoke loudly from heaven, whereby the three men were scared to death and fell to their faces before God in the Presence of Jesus (Matthew 17:4-5).

Not knowing what spirit we are of, or the true intention of God when something happens; such is a common flaw and habitual mistake we humans tend to make when trying to perceive the meaning of something we witness or experience. Instead of humbly and patiently waiting on God for further understanding, most of us arrogantly, hastily and prematurely try to interpret an event or occurrence (which we most often do inaccurately like the disciple Peter on the mountain of transfiguration). Ultimately, a visitation of God does not occur to exalt us, but to humble and level us to the foot of the cross, whereby we can see ourselves more clearly as we truly are in God's eyes, be touched, changed, and experience transformation by the divine supernatural encounter God Almighty is sending us.

When a village of the Samaritans rejected Jesus upon His arrival, His disciples James and John responded angrily saying, "Lord, will you allow us to call fire down from heaven, and consume them as Elijah did?" (Luke 9:52-54).

Jesus rebuked His disciples James and John saying, "You do not know what manner of spirit you are of" (Luke 9:55). This is because Jesus, "the Son of man, did not come to destroy men's lives, but rather to save them" (Luke 9:56). Therefore Jesus and His disciples departed and went to another village.

God Almighty promised the nation of Israel and the Jews prophetically (and we who are in Christ by faith - see Romans 11:22-27, Galatians 3:29) to bring us into our own land, cleanse us, and give us a new heart by the power of the Holy Spirit that rose Jesus Christ (the Jewish Messiah) from the dead (read Ezekiel 36:24-26; Romans 8:11,16), whereby internally God's people will be harnessed and happily constrained to yield to His Holy Spirit compelling us to obey His Word, ways and holy statutes to direct us in His blessings (verse 27).

Often times what we most need is a change in perspective, vision and outlook on life. If we are continually rubbing people the wrong way, unable to connect and get along with others, consistently full of strife within our soul; quite possibly the problem is not with others, but resident within us.

Sometimes we feel dead within and are desperately in need of divine resurrection power and a prophetic word from heaven to shake and awake us. Other times we may be outwardly bound and ensnared, whereby we need God's family of faith to intervene and send someone to help us.

Lazarus, the disciple whom Jesus loved and wept for, was wrapped in morgue clothes, prior to Jesus and His disciples coming to liberate Lazarus and let him go. Nevertheless, Jesus (God in the flesh among humanity - John 1:1,14) did not free Lazarus, but instead told His disciples to liberate and let him go (Jesus teaching His people their authority in Him when they exercise their faith and spiritual authority to step forth and speak His Word to humanity).

Jesus called Lazarus forth from the dead to return to the earth to fulfill his divine destiny (John 11:43). However upon coming back to life and returning, Lazarus was still bound with grave clothes put upon him by men at the morgue.

Beware of letting dead people, or those who work among the dead (with a deadly mindset) touch you. The putrid smell of death and a deadly toxic mindset can poison and pollute your soul, prematurely killing you prior to you fulfilling your God given destiny.

After having brought Lazarus back to life, Jesus let His disciples in on the action to fully liberate, restore and transform Lazarus. Christ's disciples took the bandages of death and preservation off Lazarus so he could breathe and fully be that which Jesus had intended for him to step into (John 11:44).

Don't prematurely prepare and rush ahead for your own funeral. Fully live your life in God and fulfill your divine destiny boldly, wholeheartedly and entirely before you cross the other side and step into eternity.

The Pharisee Saul was persecuting and killing Christians who called upon and preached Christ. When Saul had a supernatural encounter with Jesus, Saul was struck with blindness for three days (Acts 9:1-9).

Ananias, a devout disciple of Jesus Christ, came to Saul, visited and called him "Brother Saul" before praying for Saul and seeing God supernaturally restore Saul's sight (Acts 9:17-18), after which Saul was baptized. Saul would later have his named changed by God to Paul (the latter meaning "small," "humble," or "strength in God"), after which Paul entered his apostleship and ministry to the Gentiles (whom he formerly persecuted and killed). This was a remarkable supernatural transformation indeed indicative and representative of what God can miraculously do in the lives of ordinary humans who dare to believe in an extraordinary God.

Truly God did a quick and miraculous work in the life and transformation of Saul to Paul. The apostle Paul had Ananias come pray for him and remove his blindness, after which his eyesight was restored (Acts 9:17-18). It is not by chance God used Ananias to pray for murderous Saul prior to his transformation to the apostle Paul, because Ananias was esteemed by Saul to be "a devout man according to the Judaic law, having a good report among all the Jews" (Acts 22:11-13). Thus when Ananias shared his testimony about Saul's transformation, many believed and turned to Christ, being amazed at the wonderful works of God.

As the former Saul and transformed apostle Paul eloquently stated, sometimes God allows a season of suffering in order to crucify our flesh and awaken our spirit to its need for divine intervention and salvation. This is orchestrated by God "so that the spirit might be saved" (1Corinthians 5:5). Though the sufferings of this time and world seem painful and grievous, compared to the light and length of eternity, the mercy of God can be seen therein to ensure a limited amount of suffering and a greater magnitude of rejoicing and glory.

The transformed apostle Paul, the minister and ambassador of Christ's grace to the Gentiles therefore concluded: "I reckon that the sufferings of this present time are not worthy to be compared with the glory which shall be revealed in us (Romans 8:18). Paul counted all his affliction to be endured for the comfort, consolation and salvation of those to whom God called and would send him (see 2Corinthians 1:6-7). The prophet Isaiah was called by God to comfort His people scattered throughout Israel (Isaiah 40:1). God the Father, Jesus Christ the Son and the blessed Holy Spirit therefore want to call, welcome, and comfort weary humanity (see Matthew 11:28; John 14:26).

Likewise the apostle Peter who walked closely with Jesus for three years, denied Christ, and then wholeheartedly returned to his Lord and Savior weeping with tears and standing forth thereafter to preach the power of the resurrection with great boldness declared that he rejoiced whenever given opportunity to partake in Christ's sufferings, that, when His glory shall be revealed, he may be glad also with exceeding joy (1Peter 4:13). Thus Peter knew very well that suffering with Christ Jesus brings us closer to Him and the blessed Presence of the Holy Spirit, which always eventually arises mightily to show up, show off, and to turn persecution upside down into a mighty platform to preach the Good News of the glorious Gospel to the people and nations of the world for God's glory and humanity's transformation and adoption into the family of faith and God (1Peter 5:1). So remember in all times of suffering, true joy and the greatest happiness is found in the Presence of God (Psalm 16:11), the Comforter which is the blessed Holy Spirit (John 14:26) being in and with all believers (John 14:16-17) and continually coming upon us (Acts 1:8) as we step forth to be a witness of the risen Christ, so other souls among humanity can also hear the glorious Good News, partake and taste the power of the resurrection and the eternal world to come (Hebrews 6:4-5).

Thus suffering (though we resist and dislike it) is a part of life and that which makes us more like Christ. Moreover when we suffer as a Christian, in as much as we do, we too shall rejoice when the glory of God is revealed (1Peter 4:13) and suffering is turned inside out and God miraculous vindicates us, avenges our enemies and lifts us up to where we belong if we will hold our peace and let the Lord God Almighty fight our battles (Exodus 14:13; 2Chronicles 20:17; Psalm 18; 46:10).

Showing heart therefore is vitally important to live a good, purposeful, strong and meaningful life. The Bible tells us to guard our HEART with all diligence (Proverbs 4:23), from which flow the issues and insights of life. Thus heart and emotional intelligence provides us far more intuition and revelation than being merely top-heavy and intellectual (1Corinthians 2:14).

Jesus said, "in your patience, possess your soul" (Luke 21:19). Thus we must be patient with ourselves and not in such a hurry; as the purification and transformation process takes time and does not haphazardly occur overnight. We did not muddy and mess up our lives in an instant. It took time to soil and defile ourselves. Likewise the renovation, reconstruction and renewal process will take time to undergo and go through fully.

Christ warned His disciples, "in this world you will have tribulation, but be of good cheer; I have overcome the world" (John 16:33). Surely there will be many opportunities to overcome adversity and difficulties in your body, family, community, country, and in pursuit of your career and fulfillment of your destiny. Just be patient, possess your soul, and stay solid on the inside (while chaos and turbulence rages on the outside). God by the Holy Spirit will give you peace, comfort, wise counsel and courage along the way through the process.

HEART is where resurrection power first occurs, as we recognize within who God is and how God is up to something good, as in every situation He has a divine plan to show up, show off and show Himself strong in our midst (if we will hold our peace, remain calm, possess our soul, hold our tongue and wait patiently for God to step forth and show Himself in every circumstance, tribulation and test of life). As we do, today's test(s) ultimately becomes tomorrow's testimony as God Almighty miraculously intervenes and rewrites our life story, turning all things around and together for our good (Romans 8:28).

HEART is where we gain the ability to stand strong, endure hardness as good soldiers of Christ, persevere through the difficulties of life, not abandon our family and loved ones in their darkest hour and time of need, stand by people when they are at their worst and bleed, and supernaturally with divine ability access and bring forth God's love, wisdom and power to illuminate, lighten and impart resurrection life to the hopeless in dire and desperate situations.

HEART enables to endure persecution, false accusations, misinformation, misinterpretation of our motives and communication, and smear campaigns laden with mischaracterizations of who we truly are as a person. Jesus while being delivered to Pontius Pilate to be crucified recognized, Pilate would not have the power to crucify Him were it not for the fact the heavenly Father allowed and orchestrated it (John 19:11); Pilate merely being a pawn on God's divine chess board and part of our Creator and Father's divine strategy throughout the ages to send His Son Jesus to die for the sins of the world and forever liberate humanity to reconcile and restore their relationship to God (by moving their sins separating them from their heavenly Father, out of the way).

Once reconciled to God who is LOVE (1John 4:8), our heart can be awakened, washed and renewed in God's love (Romans 5:5) as the Holy Spirit who raised Christ Jesus from the dead comes to live big in us (Romans 8:11,15), healing us within and enabling us to taste and fully experience the love of God as we connect with our heavenly Father, Creator, and the blessed Holy Spirit comforts and heals us within (John 14:26). Thereafter naturally as we abide in the divine vine of love (John 15:4-5); we can begin to live by the Spirit (Galatians 5:25), renew our minds (Romans 12:1-2), be heavenly minded (Romans 8:6; Isaiah 55:8-9), and let the Holy Spirit lead and guide us into all truth (Romans 8:14; John 16:12-13). Then we can harness and put our fleshly in the backseat (Romans 8:13), as we allow the spirit within communing with God's Holy Spirit (Romans 8:16) to lead and guide us, renew our mind, and lead us with a heavenly HEART connected with and mindful of God in all things.

Prayer For Divine Oil to Awaken the Heart

Pray with me now please and SAY THIS PRAYER OUT LOUD here below to God our Father and the Lord Jesus Christ.

"Heavenly Father, thank you for sending Your only begotten Son Jesus Christ to earth to die for me. Thank you Jesus for living on earth selfishly and sacrificially, showing humanity the way, a better way, to live victoriously over the flesh, mental and physical challenges of life, relational and occupational difficulties, and unforeseeable and overwhelming circumstances that can cause and bring anguish to our hearts and souls. Give me such a HEART and spiritual power to do the same."

"Dear Jesus, as He who overcame the flesh and carnal mind, even to the extent of being crucified at Golgotha, the place of the skull, when you went to Calvary and died on the cross for me; please empower me by the blessed Holy Spirit. Send forth the Holy Spirit that rose you mightily from the dead to come live big in me and make my life what it ought to be. Come blessed and sweet Spirit of the living God to cleanse, wash, renew, restore, rejuvenate, revive, reform and revolutionize my life. Start by giving me a NEW HEART and fresh start in Jesus Name."

"Come blessed Holy Spirit in Jesus Name. Dear Jesus and heavenly Father, cleanse me with Christ's holy blood, shed on the cross for the sins of humanity. Come wonderful Savior and merciful Deliverer. Heal, help and hasten me in your grip of grace to keep and move me into the will of God. Turn my life around for the better, as the world turns daily and revolves around the sun; make my life revolve around the living God and impart newness of life within me and lift me up to live with spiritual life, divine compassion and heart. Help me to experience new life and a brand new start. I love you heavenly Father, wonderful Jesus my Savior, and blessed Holy Spirit. Take my life now and make it what you want it to be, for your glory. Give me a NEW HEART, fresh start, and rewrite my life story. Amen."

Please email me your testimony, what you felt from God when praying this prayer and reading my book (any divine Presence, internal shift, awakening, revelation, renewal, breakthrough and deliverance from evil and harmful mindsets). May God richly bless and be with you!

RevivingNations@yahoo.com

Going Deeper in Prayer

For those who dare to go deeper in prayer, beyond praying in your native tongue, God Almighty supernaturally will impart within you by the Holy Spirit a divine tongue (words that cannot be clearly articulated or uttered, but rather groanings and expressions unctioned and ushered forth by the Holy Spirit).

Jesus said, "Rivers of living water will flow forth from our belly by the Holy Spirit" (John 7:37-39). The prophet Isaiah declared: "With stammering lips and another tongue will God speak to His people. To whom He said, 'This is the rest wherewith you may cause the weary to rest; and this is the refreshing" (Isaiah 28:11-12).

The apostle Paul mentioned the Holy Spirit prays the perfect prayer according to the will of God for us, which is accomplished and performed via groanings and indiscernible utterances by the Holy Spirit, as we yield to what God stirs and erupts from within and release what we feel and hear to express ourselves to God in prayer and co-labor with the Holy Spirit in intercession to birth in our lives and the earth what God ultimately desires.

"The Holy Spirit also helps us in the midst of our infirmities: for we do not always know what we should pray for as we ought: but the Spirit itself makes intercession for us with groanings which cannot be uttered. And God that searches the hearts knows what is the mind of the Spirit, because He makes intercession for the saints according to the will of God" (Romans 8:26-27).

Although most Christians know the following verse, which says: "We know that all things work together for good to them that love God, to them who are the called according to God's purpose" (Romans 8:28); they forget that spiritual prayers in the Holy Ghost often precede the coming about of such good things from God, as prayer brings God's heavenly desires down to earth to manifest in our midst (as our prayerful demand meets divine supply) and enable us to walk in the fullness of the blessing of Christ.

When we pray in the Holy Ghost in tongues, we build ourselves up within spiritually (Jude 1:20). Remember, God is not a brain, but rather a divine Spirit (John 4:24). Therefore God's ways, methods and thoughts are higher than ours as humans (see Isaiah 55:8-9).

Jesus said, "These signs shall follow them that believe; in My Name shall they cast out devils; they shall speak with new tongues; and they shall lay hands on the sick and they shall recover" (Mark 16:17-18).

I have ministered throughout the world to Muslims, Buddhists, Hindus and Christians of all denominations worldwide and seen repeatedly God move supernaturally when I began praying in tongues.

For example in Myanmar (Asia), when I began praying in tongues among Baptists at a Bible College, suddenly all present began rolling with holy laughter, uncontrollably and unstoppably. It was a wonder to behold, experience and see.

In Cuba, (where I went illegally through Mexico, during the President Clinton administration economic embargo), when I began praying in tongues with a small group of believers inside a small building one evening; a grandmother fell straight backward on a concrete floor, passing out like a dead woman.

Although I myself as the visiting minister was a bit concerned, I heard the Holy Spirit within to tell me to relax and assured me it was the touch of God's Spirit on the woman and that she would be alright. Indeed when the grandmother got up off the concrete floor, she gave an amazing testimony about her supernatural encounter and experience with Jesus. Thus I have learned to make way, get out of the way, humbly yield, and give place to the remarkable Holy Spirit and God's miraculous work that deeply touches and transforms humanity.

Truly "the kingdom of God is not in word, but in power" (1Corinthians 4:20). The power of Almighty God is irrefutable, indisputable and inescapable - a true marvel to behold and miraculously experience as a result of Christ's mercy and blood sacrifice on the cross at Calvary for the sins, forgiveness, liberation and deliverance of humanity.

After the crucifixion and resurrection of Christ, Jesus ascended to heaven and sat down at the right hand of God the Father, after which He sent the Holy Spirit to earth to cover and empower His apostles and disciples in Jerusalem (Acts 2).

When the Holy Spirit came from heaven with the power of a rushing mighty wind and force of fire that consumes and ignites believers with zeal and passion; suddenly all the followers and believers in Christ present were supernaturally filled with the Holy Ghost and began to speak with other tongues, as the Spirit gave them utterance (Acts 2:1-4).

Jesus Himself groaned in the Spirit, another way to describe and express what the apostle Paul called speaking in tongues. Jesus groaned in the spirit prior to raising Lazarus from the dead (John 11:33-45). Thus the supernatural operations and manifestations of the Holy Spirit can produce divine healing, deliverance and resurrect the dead. Jesus so believed in the power of the resurrection by the blessed Holy Spirit, that Christ told His disciples to go forth into all the world and preach the Good News of the Gospel (Mark 16:15-20), cast out devils, heal the sick, and to raise the dead (Matthew 10:8). In fact, Jesus told His disciples they would perform greater miracles than He did (John 14:12) once Jesus returned to heaven and sent the power of the Holy Spirit, which was ultimately the Source to Jesus' success throughout His earthly ministry.

The apostle Paul, who wrote two-thirds of the New Testament and was a theologian to theologians said, "I thank God I speak with more tongues than you all" (1Corinthians 14:18) and told the churches to whom he ministered to not forbid speaking in tongues (1Corinthians 14:39). Furthermore, Paul not only prayed in tongues, but also sang in tongues, which he called praying (or singing) in the Spirit (see 1Corinthians 14:15). In other words, Paul prayed in Greek and Hebrew, but also prayed in tongues. Paul sang in Greek and Hebrew, but also sang in tongues; thereby giving birth to moves of the Holy Spirit through his prayers, worship and praise toward God. We therefore should do likewise and follow the apostle Paul as he followed Christ, he having seen and personally encountered Jesus in a miraculous way.

Join me in a time of prayer via a church service in Buenos Aires, Argentina where I was praying in tongues for people of all ages, and many were powerfully touched by the blessed and most wonderful Holy Spirit. I was only the donkey and instrument God used that night to pray for the people, but it was not me producing the supernatural, but rather the blessed Holy Spirit.

As you watch, keep an open heart and mind, ask the Holy Spirit to fill and baptize you with fresh fire (the oil of heaven to heal, liberate and free your heart) and the supernatural power that rose Christ from the dead so you can experience a new heart within and be a witness of the resurrection power of Jesus Christ in the earth to humanity (Acts 1:8).

Enter into the Presence of the Holy Spirit, our merciful and mighty Lord and Redeemer now and let the Holy Spirit fill and move in and through you from this day forward in Jesus mighty, merciful and matchless Name!

Supernatural Power Baptism in Holy Spirit Fire Miracles

https://www.youtube.com/watch?v=WxchAs2kK8c&t=1s

Enjoy and enter into the Presence of the Holy Spirit as you forget yourself, pray, welcome Jesus our Savior and the promised blessing of the Holy Spirit that Christ promised would be "in," "with," (John 14-16-17) and come "on" you to empower you to be a divine witness of Jesus to humanity (Acts 1:8).

Enjoy the passion of Christ and the unstoppable fire and fervor of the Holy Spirit (Luke 3:16). Email me your testimony as you enter into pray with me and yield to the Holy Spirit from this day forward. Invite me to your city to birth the waves of revival, call down from heaven fresh fire, awake your families and community, move people Godward, plunder hell and populate heaven as we save souls, seek and save the lost, heal the sick, deliver the bound, rejoice and make a joyful sound, and abound triumphant in the blessing of the Lord God Almighty our Redeemer.

Only believe and put feet to your faith; for surely as you do, you shall see and fully experience the glory of God (see John 11:40; James 2:26; Hebrews 11:6). In Jesus Name, I declare a new heart, new day, new way, new blessings and breakthroughs to overtake your life and lift you up to where you belong to glorify the living God.

Sources:

Wizard of Oz (1939). Gifts to scarecrow, tin man and the lion.

https://www.youtube.com/watch?v=_iRpd6PgdLI

The Wizard Of Oz (1939 Film)

https://en.wikipedia.org/wiki/The_Wizard_of_Oz_(1939_film)

If I Only Had A Heart - Wizard of Oz

https://www.youtube.com/watch?v=PU_QsEnogTg

Heart Surgery in India for $1,583 Costs $106,385 in U.S.

https://www.bloomberg.com/news/articles/2013-07-28/heart-surgery-in-india-for-1-583-costs-106-385-in-u-s-

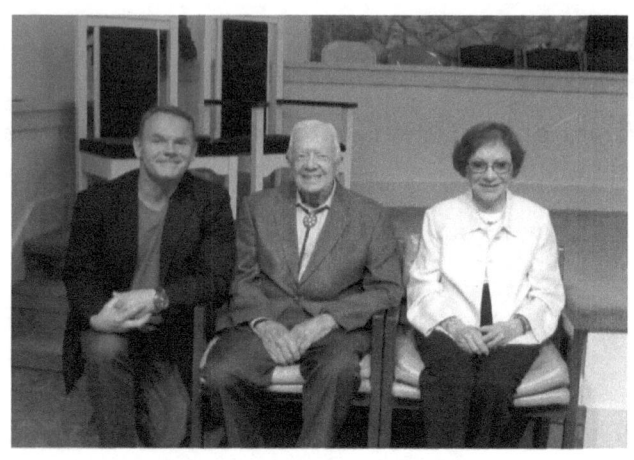

Paul with former United States President

Jimmy Carter and his wife Rosalynn

Paul F. Davis is a Worldwide Motivational Speaker who has touched 89 nations speaking for and inspiring the U.S. Military, Companies, Cruise Lines at Sea, Colleges and Universities throughout the globe.

Paul is a College and Career Counselor who has worked at Texas A&M International University and for the American China Exchange Society. Paul has earned 4 Master degrees with the highest honors from the University of Texas (Educational Leadership), New York University (Global Affairs), Michigan State College of Law (Global Food Law), the University of Alabama (Health). Paul completed his training in College Counseling with the University of California at Los Angeles.

Paul is the author of more than 70 books including:

- Breakthrough For A Broken Heart
- Energized by Anger
- Angry at God and Everyone Else
- Update Your Identity
- Integrity of Heart
- Wealthy Mind
- Empowering & Liberating Women To Achieve Greatness
- Healthy Relationships
- Dating, Relationships, Love and Marriage
- College Match & Self-Discovery
- Educational Leadership and School Instructional Improvement
- College Admissions Secrets & Interview Strategies
- Charter Schools: Faith, Free Choice and Inferior Education for Profit Preying on Minorities
- United States of Arrogance
- The Future of Food
- Geostrategy to Protect Environmental Health & Food Security

Many more books and videos can be seen at Paul's website below. Please also connect with Paul via social media.

www.PaulFDavis.com

www.Linkedin.com/in/worldproperties

www.Facebook.com/speakers4inspiration

www.Twitter.com/PaulFDavis

RevivingNations@yahoo.com